And the
BEST DIET
is...

DR. F. HAMILTON
Bariatric Surgeon

HIGH BRIDGE BOOKS
HOUSTON

Contents

Introduction

As a bariatric surgeon and an obesity medicine physician, I had people constantly asking which diets are the best. In my practice, I have heard it all—water-only diets, cabbage soup diets, colonic cleanse diets, you name it. This book was partly inspired by my patients. As they asked me about diets, I felt it was my duty to dig into the science and data behind the diets. I did not want to offer my patient just another "fad diet." I wanted to give them something that would really help.

Believe it or not, we do not learn about nutrition in medical school. I heard that they offer a course on it now, but when I was in medical school, we did not even get one full class about nutrition. We learned about how the body acts and responds, but our focus was mostly on how the body works, not what to feed it. I went through my entire residency learning the minimal about nutrition. Yes, we learned about the building blocks of nutrition like protein, fats and carbohydrates, and other minerals but nothing about diets.

During my fellowship, I trained with an obesity medicine doctor, and when we were not operating or seeing surgical patients, I would volunteer to sit and learn from her. I think she is a pivotal reason why I became so interested in bariatric surgery, which also includes nutrition. When I started my practice and wanted to learn more about the medicine of bariatrics, learning about diets among several other things was a top priority. After all, your diet is one of the simplest changes you can make and can help you live a much longer life. Remember, there is no cure for some illnesses, such as COVID-19, and if you want to increase your chances for survival, a proper diet is one of the easiest ways to do that.

I also learned that people who did the best made permanent changes in their diet. As many of us know, surgery alone is not the answer, although many people still lost weight eating the same after surgery. Those bad eating habits and their weight loss only lasted so long, and then, like many other things, it caught back up to them and the weight returned. I have seen people just eat better and lose the weight with no surgery or exercise, and I have also seen people diet for months with no results.

I wanted to research whether a better diet truly existed. I wrote this book not only to educate and inform but also to have everything in one place. There are several books on keto, paleo, or intermittent fasting, but I wanted to put the most important aspects of each popular diet people ask about into one book.

With, the current diet culture, and the obsession with healthy eating at the forefront, opens the door to another problem—fad diets.

These are the diets you see all over social media, the diets usually plastered on top of normal foods to make them seem healthier. "Keto bread" or "Paleo pancake mix," for example, is prevalent in our grocery stores, so do these labels mean anything?

What are some of the fad diets, and do they help you or are they just popular? Why do they take up space on our favorite foods? Are they really better than your current food choices?

Well, fad diets can be just that: fads. They're what everyone's going crazy about and paying attention to at the moment, but in reality, they have some downsides and risks. I thought it was important to investigate the fad diets as well as their pros and cons. I also wanted to research what the best diet is or if that even exists.

We will answer many of those questions in this book. We'll discuss in detail the fad diets and what they are. We'll tackle the most popular dietary options and go over the pros and cons, what you can and can't eat, and the benefits and drawbacks of each. At the end of each chapter, we'll also talk about the bottom line and whether it's right for you.

If you're sick of digging through and trying to figure out whether keto or Mediterranean is right for you or not, then look no further. We'll give you the big picture and offer you a chance to fully understand exactly what each diet has to offer.

1

The Low-Carb Diet

Let's begin by discussing one of the most popular diets that doctors recommend and that many people are on—the low-carb diet. The low-carb diet—and, in particular, the ketogenic diet—is one of the most popular fad diets on the market today. It has been modified in many versions, but we will discuss the overview here. A ketogenic diet is an extremely low-carb diet, where you're only eating about 20 grams of carbs a day.

The science behind this is simple. Our bodies use carbohydrates (carbs) to fuel up, similar to putting gas in a car. Carbs, however, are a temporary fuel source, and usually after consuming carbs, our blood sugar spikes. Keto, otherwise known as the ketogenic diet, encourages you to eat fewer carbs, reducing your carb intake to almost nothing. The purpose is to deplete your carbohydrate stores so ketones, which are produced via ketosis, are formed and burned as an energy source.

Are Ketones Good for You?

You might wonder if ketones are a valuable source of energy. Well, they are. Ketones are an alternative to glucose.

When you don't eat as many carbs, your liver produces ketones; these come from fat.

Ketones provide a fuel source for the body and are great for brain health and development. The brain is very hungry, and it requires a lot of energy, so it needs either glucose (which comes in carbohydrates consumed) or ketones.

On keto, your entire body switches from mostly glucose as a supply of fuel to fat as a supply, and you become a fat-burning machine.

The fat burns much faster once your insulin levels completely drop. You'll shed the fat on your body, thereby losing weight.

Not only is this good for losing weight, but it offers some benefits you may otherwise not get from your regular diet. In the next section, we will discuss different versions of some of the popular low-carb and keto diets.

The Atkins Diet

Let's review other popular versions of keto diets before we get into the actual pros and cons of the current ketogenic diet. Many people think Atkins and keto are the same diet, but we'll highlight what the Atkins diet is and how it is different.

The Atkins diet was originally promoted by Dr. Robert C. Atkins, who wrote a best-selling book about it in 1972. The Atkins diet doesn't involve calorie counting or controlling portions, but it requires you to track your carbs, just like with keto. However, there is a difference here.

The Atkins diet focuses on getting your protein in first, then fat and low net carbs, where keto focuses on eating more healthy fats, then protein and very low-carb. Atkins uses something called net carbs. Now, what's that? It's basically the total carbs minus the fiber content. So let's say you eat a half cup of broccoli, and that's 2.3 grams of carbs. But you're not actually eating 2.3 grams of carbs—1.3 grams of that is fiber, which is absorbed by the digestive system and later expelled.

The net carbs are 1 gram.

The idea is to eat fewer net carbs while also incorporating exercising to feel good. You can have carbs, but the purpose is to control blood sugar and from there burn off the fat stores in the body, while also keeping you nice and full.

We all have a carb tolerance, something we can achieve that won't force us to lose or gain weight. Your tolerance might be higher than your friends', which is fine. But once you've lost the weight, you then want to figure out this tolerance to maintain it.

With Atkins, you should exercise, but it isn't vital and required. The Atkins diet has phases, as outlined below:

- Phase 1 (induction): Under 20 grams of carbs per day for two weeks. Eat high-fat, high-protein, with low-carb vegetables like leafy greens. This kick-starts weight loss.
- Phase 2 (balancing): Slowly add more nuts, low-carb vegetables, and small amounts of fruit back to your diet.
- Phase 3 (fine-tuning): When you're very close to your goal weight, add more carbs to your diet until weight loss slows down.
- Phase 4 (maintenance): Here, you can eat as many healthy carbs as your body can tolerate

without regaining weight up to 100 grams of net carbs. But this requires tracking your net carb count daily with every meal.

The last part of this diet might seem cumbersome. After all, who wants to count carbs till the end of their days? You don't have to sit there tabulating everything till the cows come home, but you must monitor how many carbs you can have without gaining weight.

How does Atkins compare to just a low-carb diet? Atkins is one of the most popular forms of low-carb dieting next to keto, and it was *the* low-carb diet before keto became popular. Atkins has many plans, but they all involve one specific part—low carbs, a modest amount of protein, and a lot of fats. Atkins has dietary restrictions besides just low net carbs, and unlike low-carb only or keto, the carb allowance grows with time.

With keto and other low-carb diets, your carb count is very restricted until you go off the diet. Another difference with Atkins is you don't just stay with a small amount of carbs; it increases as needed until you hit 100 grams a day. The Atkins diet pushes for 30 percent of your calories to be from protein no matter what phase you're in, whereas purely low-carb diets are more focused on the carb restriction.

For a balanced diet, the FDA recommends that 10 to 35 percent of your calories to be from protein, whereas in Atkins, it starts at 30 percent. Atkins is much more flexible in the foods you can eat when compared to keto, and this is often considered the less restrictive of the two diets.

The South Beach Diet

Another popular diet labeled keto or low-carb is the South Beach Diet, which was created in 2003 by a cardiologist named Arthur Angaston. This is a modified version of the low-carb diet. You essentially want to lower the carbs and have more protein. But this diet doesn't have stringent guidelines like the other ones, and it isn't strictly low-carb either.

There is a keto version where you eat very few carbs, but it's not as popular. The idea is to balance out the carbs, proteins, and fats, making sure that you eat lots of fiber. You want to eat foods with complex carbs, and you don't eat simple carbs like sugary foods and baked goods. In other words, lay off the sweets, but if you want a little bit of beans, go for it.

With this diet, you can eat legumes, whole grains, and even beans and fruit. This one wants you to learn about the different kinds of fats, pushing you to eat more monosaturated fats, which are considered healthy fats, and not a ton of saturated or even trans fats.

Mostly, you want to keep the carb intake at around 28 percent. So it's not a ton, but again, you're not cutting carbs cold turkey like you would with keto.

For reference, the average person consumes 225–325 grams of carbs before beginning the diet and then limits the carbs to 140 grams. This might be restricted to 40–50 grams of carbs for the keto version.

Those are some of the differences, so how does this diet work? Well, it also has phases.

In the first phase, you cut out all carbs and don't drink juice and alcohol. You eat more lean protein and soy products. You'll also eat high-fiber veggies along with un-saturated fats. This happens during the first two weeks of this diet, and as a result, they say you can lose up to 13 pounds.

In the second phase, you begin to add things back slowly, including pasta, brown rice, veggies, and fruits. This results in one to two pounds lost a week mostly, creating a steady, simple weight loss.

The third and final phase is maintenance, where you learn to limit the carbs you have and instead enjoy a life-style that works for you and is healthy too!

So in general, the grams are broken down per phase in the following way:

- 20–40 grams for phase 1
- 40–100 in phase 2
- Up to 140 in phase 3

If you're starting the South Beach Diet, you're eating about half of what you were in carbs. It is also a way to re-strict your diet and learn to eat better. It might not seem fun at first, but again, this weight loss diet has worked for many people.

What About Just Low-Carb Diets?

Low-carb diet plans are similar to both keto and Atkins. At-kins restricts carbs to up to 100 grams, but with low-carb, you choose how much you will restrict.

You want to slowly lower how many carbs you con-sume so you can stay satiated and also lose weight. You can eat carbs, but you don't eat a ton of them. The purpose of a low-carb diet is mostly to lose weight and improve your health, and this has been in use for decades. It's often recommended by doctors, and I will admit I was one of those doctors. I feel there is a time for eating lower carbs, but as I have learned and grown, I realized it is about what you eat and the type of carbs being eaten, not just lowering the total carbs.

On any low-carb diet you lose weight, and your markers are better not just because it is a keto or Atkins diet but because you are changing certain aspects of your regular diet. You are ultimately eating better because you are paying more attention to what you are eating But I do not want to give too much away this early in the book. Let's keep learning.

The cool thing about doing just a low-carb diet is that you work to restrict your carbs a little without worrying about calories. Low-carb offers more freedom to consume what you want to consume, but also restrict the carbs to help you gradually lose weight and improve your overall health.

You're eating the same things as on keto, but without the severe restriction, and eating healthy amounts of protein and fats. You may also eat some vegetables you may not have on keto since they are higher in carbs. You eat till you're full, and you don't have to worry about calorie counting or even complex weighing. You also don't need to overly track your macros like you do with keto and Atkins.

A Summary of the Popular Low-Carb Diets:

You probably aren't sure of the differences or need a simplified explanation of the three modified diets discussed in this keto section—Atkins, South Beach, and low-carb. They all are similar and are all low-carb versions of one another. They all whistle the same tune of "eat fewer carbs, eat more fat and protein," but there are differences, as follows:

- Keto: Up to 20–25 grams of carbs, severe carb restriction. You eat a lot of fat and moderate protein
- Atkins: You eat up to 100 grams of carbs when in the maintenance phase. You can eat a lot of protein and a moderate amount of fat
- South Beach: At the lowest, you take in 40–50 grams of carbs on the keto side, up to 140 grams during the maintenance period. You eat anywhere from 45–65 percent of your calories in carbs after you finish phase 1, so much less carb-restricted
- Low-carb: You choose how to restrict your carbs and essentially eat more fats and proteins and restrict carb-rich food

The first two require a little more monitoring of what you eat, while the third is a good starting point for those just interested in eating less carbohydrates and eating healthier.

2

Let's Discuss the Skinny on Keto

When we talk about how keto works, it usually involves a severe carb restriction. But what are the actual figures? Well, for starters, on keto, only 5 percent of calories come from carbs as compared to the normal recommendation of 45–65 percent of calories coming from carbs. These include low-carb veggies and leafy greens. For the most part, you don't have fruits, starchy veggies, or even whole grains and beans. Twenty percent of your calories in a keto diet should come from proteins (slightly less than in Atkins), including meat, cheese, and eggs. The rest comes from fats, and this includes fatty oils, nuts, butter, and avocados. The key here is healthy fats.

At first, this differs greatly from what you're used to, but to cut the carbs enough to burn ketones, you must restrict carb intake within these guidelines. Mostly, your body turns these carbs into glucose, and when you cut that out, it forces ketones from the liver to be produced and used. You need to do this for about three weeks before ketosis kicks in.

What Are the Pros of Keto?

What are the benefits of keto? It has many benefits. The first is, of course, weight loss. People lose a lot of weight and often will drop that weight quicker than they would not on a keto diet. But it's more than that. They don't feel as hungry, and many report eating less than they normally do. Fat keeps a person fuller than if they have just eaten a high-carb diet.

Weight loss comes from ketosis itself, but because you naturally restrict your carbs and eat less by limiting some food groups, you also won't be eating nearly as many calories as you normally would. Another benefit is that you can have those high-fat foods you otherwise may not enjoy, such as fatty fish, meats, nuts, butter, and even cheese. You can do this all while losing weight too!

For some people, it offers another benefit as well. Those with epilepsy also notice they have fewer seizures when doing keto. Bodybuilders and athletes also might use it to help trim up and reduce their fat in a shorter time. This diet has also been shown to help those with neurological conditions such as Parkinson's, but there aren't enough benefits to either confirm or deny this claim.

Many also report they have better energy levels, and this may be because you won't feel randomly tired after eating dinner on keto because there is no carb crash. When your body gets used to not eating carbs all the time on the keto diet, not only will you feel less hungry, but you also won't feel the sugar spikes and drops that normally come. This is great if you're looking to stay focused and alert. And I feel that the ketones from fatty acids crossing the blood-brain barrier help with the disorders of the brain, such as

ADHD, Parkinson's, and seizures. This is due to the high fatty acids that often result from taking high doses of omega often recommended for those disorders.

Some patients also report better blood glucose levels, and it also helps curb insulin resistance. So for diabetics, this can be a great diet to help control their blood sugar. Of course, you can do that with other low-carb diets, but if you have issues controlling your sugar or experience high levels of insulin resistance, this can help immensely. Not only that, but keto can also help with lowering your cholesterol levels, help reduce symptoms of Alzheimer's, and has even been shown to slow its progression.

A ketogenic diet can help with PCOS, help reduce the instance of concussions, and can help with brain injuries too. Again, this mechanism is due to the higher intake of omega 3s and healthy fats. Some even reported it helps with acne since you're eating less processed foods and sugars.

Of course, it also provides the benefits of a healthy diet and lifestyle. Many like it because it gets them to eat right and eat less carb-ridden food. You naturally have better appetite control, and you'll notice your hunger pangs decrease a lot over time. You can also pair keto with intermittent fasting as well to enhance the efforts to reverse your diabetes or to help you lose weight. You don't have to mix this with the fasting diets. You also might notice that you're saving money by snacking less. Many report they only need to eat twice a day on keto, which is remarkably different from other eating styles.

Your blood sugar will thank you too. If you're prediabetic, have metabolic syndrome, which is pre-diabetes and high cholesterol with increased abdominal girth, or you have type II diabetes, this diet can help reverse it. For those with IBS or other stomach conditions, keto is great. Stomach cramps and gas are far less when on keto than on other diets, and you might see an improvement in your IBS symptoms. The cool part about that is you notice the difference in only a day or two.

What to Eat

This all sounds good, but now you want to know what to eat on keto. We went over some things, but here's a more definitive list:

- Cooking oils such as olive and coconut oil
- Butter, especially grass-fed butter
- Ghee
- Fish and seafood
- High-protein meats, such as bison, steak, and chicken
- Cheese
- Avocadoes
- Eggplants
- Celery
- Cucumber
- Cauliflower
- Peppers
- Broccoli
- Eggs
- Seasonings of choice

There are some "keto-friendly" options of your favorite carb-rich foods, but those are a bit hit or miss on quality.

Often, the nutrients are taken out as well, which can pose a problem for some people. The big thing to remember here is that you must keep the carb intake below 50 grams for the best results.

Ideally, it should be 20 or under, but this is hard for many people. The rule of thumb is the lower the carbs, the more effective this diet can be for achieving ketosis. You'll also improve Type II diabetes and overall body weight by reducing your carbs.

Some people use keto recipes to help count carbs, but you can also use carb trackers, and manually counting carbs to help you figure out how much you've eaten.

What Not to Eat

Unfortunately, this means many foods can't be eaten as well. Here's a list of some foods you shouldn't eat:

- Fruits of any kind, minus tomatoes and avocados
- Potatoes
- Cooked pasta of any kind
- Beer
- Cooked rice and other cooked grains
- Bread, including whole wheat bread
- Sodas
- Juice
- Candy
- Chocolate
- Donuts
- Baked goods

All of these foods are loaded with carbs. You might not even realize it until you look into it, but a tiny donut puts you at your carb limit—or can be 2.5 times the ideal amount of carbs you should have on a ketogenic diet. This is a bit of a wake-up call for some people, but with many Americans dying from heart disease and diabetes, our diets need an overhaul. Another part of this keto diet—and for me, the main benefit—is avoiding highly processed foods. Processed foods have so many nutrients taken out of the food during the "process," and that also creates empty calories. The best thing to do is to eat low-processed foods and cook recipes of your own as needed.

Also, avoid anything that says "low fat." That usually means it's high in carbs. If you're unsure, check the labels on the packaging and see if you can have it. The keto diet should be somewhat high in proteins, but you need more fat than anything. Remember, protein isn't the fuel, fat is. Many low-fat products only contain carbs and don't have enough of the other nutrients.

If you're stumped on what to drink on keto, the best thing to have is water. It's an essential part of losing weight. Coffee and tea are next since they don't contain carbs unless you add sweeteners. Some milk and cream are okay, but record those carbs. And sorry, Starbuck fans, but often those lattes are off the list. Wine is the best alcoholic drink to have since it doesn't need to be mixed like others and only contains a few grams of carbs per serving depending on the wine. But remember those add up, so track even the carbs you drink, as they count toward your total carbs. Apparently, now you can get keto alcohol and keto drinks too if you want.

Keto Flu—A Common Issue

One thing that makes starting keto hard is the keto flu, which results in experiencing flu-like symptoms. You may also notice you're lethargic and your energy levels are depleted. This is a symptom of the diet working since you have far fewer stores of carbs and your body is using up everything it has. The best way to treat this is to make sure your body is getting enough fat to help reduce cravings. Sometimes, you might need to add a little more carbs to stave off keto flu.

Remember to drink enough water and get enough electrolytes as well. Keto flu lasts longer for some than others, but if you're adequately prepared to treat this, it isn't a big deal.

What Are the Cons of Keto?

What is the downside of keto? Unfortunately, this diet has a lot more cons than pros, though it sounds good on paper.

First, it's very hard to sustain long term for most people. You're restricting your diet a lot, and those restrictions are hard to stick to. This diet is good for short-term weight loss to adopt better eating habits, but it often creates a yo-yo phenomenon, where you gain all that weight back.

When you get off keto, you will probably eat those carbs once again. Unless you use the diet to adopt better eating habits, you won't lose weight. It's a fad diet because it's a temporary action and it can increase many other risks.

Ketosis itself can be very hard to achieve because you need to track everything you consume. It also is hard to tell if you're in ketosis short of a blood test or urine test. Several of my patients came in week after week testing their urine and had not obtained ketosis yet, and that only led to frustrations. One study found that keto causes the body to lose weight, but it leads to normal weight gain once you have a normal diet. It isn't an effective long-term diet.

Another downside is nutrient deficiency and calorie depletion. You won't get enough nutrients, including fiber, vitamins, and minerals. You're consuming hardly any fruits and veggies, which can cause problems. While the carb depletion feeling may be temporary because of the "keto flu," it creates other problems, including malnutrition and constipation.

It also might create a negative impact on your heart. The American Heart Association says your saturated fat intake shouldn't be over 6 percent. On keto, people are encouraged to eat fats but most rely on saturated fats. This can increase the risk for heart disease, and many report an increase in the lipids and fats after eight weeks on keto. For those with a bad heart or at risk for heart disease, this isn't a good diet.

Sometimes renal issues happen as well. Some patients with kidney disease have an increased risk of needing dialysis. That's because the more ketones in the body, the more the renal system must filter and process. Many patients also experience dehydration since the glycogen is being expelled from the body. That holds water, and it moves into the bloodstream.

Another major problem is food obsession. This is a problem for some people since you must manage all the foods you eat, tracking them left and right. It disconnects you from what your body needs, and instead, you can become obsessed with food. This can put someone at risk for eating disorders or obsessing over numbers instead of what the body wants. This is also why some people struggle with keto since they are so focused on getting X amount of carbs that they don't realize their body is starving for nutrients.

This can get so bad it can lead to distress if a person overeats or binge eats, and then they feel shame and end up purging or restricting further. This creates guilt, which leads to more restrictions. Some people develop anorexia and bulimia in some cases. It isn't a long-term diet, and many report it isn't all that good for you over time. It's a temporary solution, but it doesn't fix the problem at hand.

Is It Right for Me?

So is keto the best diet for you? I know people who have been doing keto for years and it has worked for them. But I tell my patients this diet really isn't sustainable as a lifestyle change. Mostly, it's a temporary solution to a long-term problem. Most who go on this diet are trying to lose weight. The keto diet has worked for many of my patients, but many gain it all back. It offers short-term success in reduced appetite and perhaps better blood sugars.

This diet is best for those who want to control their blood sugar better or who have type II diabetes. This is also a good diet for those with epilepsy since it can help in controlling seizures. If you want to use it as a temporary solution to lose weight, it can help, but the truth is it will not be a sustainable diet. The risks certainly outweigh the rewards. Keto is a temporary solution to a major problem, and most don't realize until it's too late that it's certainly not a sustainable means to lose fat.

And the Best Diet is...

The problem is what you're eating causes weight gain and medical problems. Yes, there must be some changes to the way you eat, but even starting to be mindful when eating can trigger this change. For people who struggle with brain disorders, as mentioned, this truly may be the better diet for them, but if that is not you, other diets may be a better fit.

3

The Paleo Diet

"Let's eat like our ancestors!" Okay, while you will not go out and hunt a deer (unless you do that for sport already), you can eat like your ancestors. That means eating the foods they ate. Although you may not gather berries—and you probably shouldn't because most of us don't know whether it's a poisonous berry or something safe—you can go to the grocery store and get these age-old paleo foods to consume. But is it worth doing?

Let's look more into the paleo diet. It's another diet heralded as a popular one to help with losing weight. But is it right for you? In this chapter, we will discuss what it is, and some aspects to better help you understand if it is the best diet for you. We'll also go over the truth behind eating like our ancestors, and whether it's something worth doing, or if it's better to stay with the diets of this century.

Overview

The idea behind the paleo diet is simple: eat the way our hunter-gatherer ancestors used to eat, rather than the processed, refined foods we have today.

Our ancestors were small, and they had to be able to move fast to get away from dangers like a mammoth or some other large creature that no longer exists today. They usually only packed on the pounds when they were getting ready for winter, which they quickly shed afterward. That was the hunter-gatherer body, and it survived for a long time.

But when sugar came along, things changed. We got potbellies, we became obese, and since then, it's become an epidemic of massive proportions.

The paleo diet looks to turn the clock back so you can eat better, and many people love this diet because you're eating right and cutting out processed foods. Most of all, you're changing your habits, so you stop eating garbage food and instead focus on whole foods that are good for you. Sugar is practically cut out from this diet minus natural fruits, as well as anything with processed chemicals.

Although it's impossible to eat exactly what our ancestors used to eat back then, the main idea behind the paleo diet is whole foods. This whole-food diet presumably helps to lower insulin levels, reduce the rate of diabetes, curb obesity, and offset heart disease. It also means losing weight without counting calories and can offer major improvements to one's health and wellness.

No One Right Way to Go Paleo

The cool thing about paleo is that it's very flexible. While there are a few basic guidelines, there isn't just one way to do paleo. It involves eating the right kinds of food that are part of the diet.

Some will eat more low-carb when doing paleo, while others will eat high-carb, but the carbs focus on plants and fruit. The idea, however, is to eat only things that are whole,

that don't have additives, artificial sweeteners, or processed chemicals. So if you love nuts and berries with fruits,
then have at it! If you can't live without your cheese and
milk, you technically can have that as well. Though many
people forgo dairy on this diet simply because it may cause
allergies, this is ultimately up to you.

Our hunter-gatherer ancestors didn't eat grains either,
and many presume the reason obesity is an epidemic is because of the addition of grains into the diet. Our former pre-
historic bodies were small and lean to help them move fast
to get away from predators and to catch prey. Once wheat
was introduced into society, the weight came on. Paleo is
like taking a time machine back to the past and eating like
they did, but with modifications as needed.

Paleo doesn't have one stringent set of guidelines either. There is no calorie or carb limit like with carb reduc-
tion diets, so for those who get obsessed and caught up in
the numbers, this could be the diet you're looking for. The
diet involves only eating certain foods and following general guidelines. With paleo, there isn't calorie counting or
macros tracking, although if you feel like you want to do
that, you're more than welcome to. It works based on the
person's needs and preferences and what provides them
with the best nutrition possible.

What to Eat on Paleo

On paleo, the parameters are generalized, and you can eat
more than you did on keto. But there are a few guidelines.
It's better to have foods that aren't filled with additives and
preservatives and are organic, grass-fed, or free-range depending on the food at hand.

A list of the types of foods is below:

- Lean cuts of chicken, beef, and pork
- Eggs
- Game animals, including venison and bison
- Fish
- Fruits, including strawberries, mangoes, cantaloupe, and others
- Non-starchy vegetables, including asparagus and pumpkin
- Nuts and seeds
- Olive oil, walnut oil, and flaxseed oil

That doesn't seem like much, but spices also offer more flavorful foods. Some people may add other little things, including protein substitutes for vegetarians. The idea is to eat foods that the paleolithic humans might've had in their diet. While we can't go back in time for confirmation, this is a good set of guidelines on what you should eat.

What Not to Eat

The paleo diet isn't super restricted, but processed foods are off the table. No cookies, no chips. Keep those for the cheat day. Similarly, butter, margarine, and sugar shouldn't be a part of the paleo diet because they are processed. Use ghee instead as a butter substitute. Now, dairy is up for debate for those on paleo. Paleo rarely includes dairy, but some people do have it. However, it usually reveals a dairy allergy. Many paleolithic humans didn't have dairy, so it's not technically part of the diet. But some will have it in moderation, or maybe they'll eliminate it to see if there is a dairy allergy.

Legumes are also off the table. They weren't accessible to these people and aren't easily digestible. But some people aren't as strict about paleo as others, so they might include dairy products and some legumes. For example, beans and peanuts may be allowed if you're not doing a restricted version of this diet. If you're a fan of beans and like to eat them, you can still incorporate them, just have a limited amount.

However, all grains are completely restricted. That's because humans didn't eat cereal grains back then, so keeping them on the list would defeat the purpose of this kind of diet. Starchy and root vegetables such as potatoes and sweet potatoes should not be consumed either. Sweets and sugars are all taken out too, including table sugar and honey. The only sweetener usually used is agave syrup, and that's in moderation. But anything processed, including deli meats and hot dogs, are also restricted.

You're limiting many of the sweets in our American diet, and processed chemicals and similar foods. While it is a bit of a shock to some people, you don't have to cut all of these cold turkey—you can slowly remove them from your diet. The beauty is that the diet is super flexible. There is room for different combinations, and that's part of the reason some like the paleo diet more than others.

For sugar substitutes, some also will use maple syrup and stevia. Dairy is usually substituted with coconut or almond milk rather than normal milk. Butter is substituted as well. Paleo might seem to have a lot of restrictions, but the goal is to go natural and eat as similar as you can to our paleolithic ancestors.

What Are the Pros of Paleo?

The paleo diet has quite a few benefits, and there's a reason many enjoy it. To begin, it balances the energy during the day, so your blood sugar isn't spiking and dropping. It's also good for those who have prediabetes since it can help control and stabilize the blood sugar. Since you're not eating or drinking as many processed and sugary items, there are fewer carbs in the body and fewer chemicals being eaten. This can lead to better skin and teeth for many people.

Because you're reducing your carb intake and eating less processed foods, you can burn off a lot of the stored fat, and it can help with creating lean tissues.

Your workouts and exercises will feel better, and they'll be more effective. The decreased sugar creates more balanced energy, offering better, more rewarding workouts.

Paleo is anti-inflammatory too since you're eating foods that contain antioxidants, which curb free radicals and inflammation. Those with inflammatory conditions also notice a change in their prevalence, as it can help curb and control those conditions in some people. It might also provide relief from diabetes, heart disease, obesity, and autoimmune conditions, which is partially attributed to the weight loss and the anti-inflammatory effects.

A big benefit many don't discuss is food allergies. Many of us might be allergic to foods and not even realize it. But paleo helps us recognize these food allergies so we can do something about them. For example, some of us don't even realize we have a dairy allergy until we remove it from our diets. By removing dairy and slowly integrating it back in, we can find that out. There are alternatives too.

The same can be said for gluten since some are allergic and may experience bloating, gas, and acne.

Paleo is good for sleeping too. Those who do paleo report better sleep patterns over time. This is partially attributed to balancing sugars and building a better, more intact circadian rhythm to feel better and create a stabilized schedule. Paleo works because the concept is simple—it involves mostly clean eating, allows us to be in better control of our lives, and allows us to eat lots of fruits and veggies. One of the best things about Paleo is that it helps us reconnect with nature by eating less processed foods. This is great for people who like to garden. Although it isn't for everyone, the diet has the potential for marked benefits.

What Are the Cons of Paleo?

Paleo sounds great, but all diets come with some cons. For starters, this obviously isn't for everyone. Since many of the food groups are eliminated (i.e., grains), this could pose a problem for procuring essential nutrients and vitamins. Some healthy food gets taken out of the diet. Many who use this diet either need a multivitamin or a calcium supplement since the lack of dairy could affect the bone density and the state of your teeth.

The lack of grains can cause a decrease in fiber, which can create issues with your gut health. You may have bad bowel movements or trouble expelling on this diet. But if you want to fix that issue, you can always take a fiber supplement or incorporate some fiber-rich veggies into your diet.

There is also the lack of legumes consumption, such as peas, lentils, and other beans. While some research shows it's okay to cut these out, it isn't necessarily a good idea since legumes contain selenium, manganese, and magnesium, which are helpful for our gut. Not only that, humans today aren't like those during the paleolithic period. We've evolved in terms of adaption to eating those foods.

While, sure, our diets could benefit from less sugar, cutting out these other healthy foods puts us at risk for nutrient deficiency. The diet also doesn't account for the wide amount of foods available then, and there isn't enough evidence to establish what truly was eaten during those ancient times, and, let's face it, certain animals they had like mammoths no longer exist today. There simply isn't evidence to fully back up that what you eat on this diet is what they were eating.

Also, the portions allowed exceed the daily allowances, so it may be too much for you. The diet isn't specifically used just to lose weight.

This diet is also very expensive because it focuses more on whole foods. You aren't shopping in the inner aisles of the store but rather the outer aisles, and you'll notice it costs more than other diets. This is especially true when trying to find paleo substitutes.

There also isn't a limit on saturated fat intake. That means the overconsumption of saturated fats is still possible, and that can account for weight gain, high blood pressure, and heart issues. So even though it's "healthy," it doesn't account for all the bad things out there.

Finally, this diet has proven to help with weight loss and such, but it doesn't have the scientific research behind it that a diet should. There isn't enough evidence this diet will help you, and we don't know how they really lived all those years ago. While, yes, it offers some benefits, our assumptions could be wrong.

And let's be honest, were hunter-gatherers the model of health? They carried a lot of parasites and were subjected to many infectious diseases, including atherosclerosis. These modern fruits and veggies also aren't like what our ancestors consumed either, so we can never fully emulate this diet. The lack of information on whether people ate like this back then, combined with there being no right way, makes it a crapshoot on whether it can be a reliable diet. Some people get benefits from cutting the bad carbs out, but by cutting grains, dairy, and legumes you are missing important vitamins and minerals.

Is it Right for Me?

It depends. Some people find this diet is great because it offers the chance to eat healthy foods. After all, the paleo diet is simple to follow and focuses on healthy foods. If you're tired of always reaching for something sweet and sugary, this is a great way to get out of that habit.

But the thing is, it's not concrete. There isn't a "can and can't eat" list. Even dairy is debatable on this diet. For some people, the restrictions on food make it a bit more "boring" than other diets. But it also doesn't involve immense amounts of calorie counting like other diets do.

If you have allergies, this is good to use because it can help pinpoint if you're just over-consuming something or if you have an allergic reaction. Many people will find out they have a dairy allergy or even a gluten allergy on this diet. It's good if you suspect that and want to know more. This diet may also be good for people with inflammatory disorders such as rheumatoid arthritis, osteoarthritis, and perhaps some autoimmune disorders such as lupus.

However, this diet necessitates the need for supplements. You're not getting enough of certain vitamins and minerals. Nutrient deficiency is a common problem on paleo, so if you choose to implement this diet, make sure you have a plan for accounting for the nutrients you're losing by switching to paleo.

This diet isn't all that good for weight loss; however, it's good if you want to practice eating right. But again, this diet isn't concrete. It involves many different factors, and many people don't realize that it may not be ideal for them. While the concept of eating these healthy foods should be considered, and perhaps curbing the sugars and processed chemicals in your diet is a good idea, the cons may outweigh the benefits since you're kicking out a couple of the major food groups, which can put you at risk for nutrient deficiency if you're not careful.

4

The Mediterranean Diet

Imagine you're sitting at a table with some of your close friends and family, passing around some lemon garlic shrimp in fettuccine while drinking some of your favorite wine with a side of salad topped with a strawberry vinaigrette. All while sitting outside, listening to the waves crashing along the shore (for added effects).

Sounds good? Well, you can get that in the Mediterranean diet. But wait, that's a bunch of carbs. Can you eat carbs on the Mediterranean diet? The answer is yes, but there are some limits. This is another popular diet, but is it right for you? Here, we'll discuss the basics of the diet, and what the different parts of the diet call for.

Overview

This diet focuses on eating traditional foods that Italy and Greece had back in 1960. They were a lot healthier than Americans, and they had a much lower risk of different lifestyle diseases, including diabetes and heart attacks. This diet has been well-researched, and many studies came out showing it not only helped with weight loss, but it can prevent strokes, type 2 diabetes, and even premature death. This diet is a lot more lenient than other diets since there isn't one right away to follow it. That's because there are many countries around that area, and every place has different foods.

It's definitely one of the less restrictive diets since you're not focusing on counting calories or carbs. Instead, you're eating foods based on what they're eating in Greece and Italy. This is considered one of the best diets for those who don't like restrictive diets. It's similar to paleo, where it's all not set in stone. Like modified paleo with dairy and grains, Mediterranean eating has some flexibility too, which is why many like it.

You can always count calories, but the focus should be on the foods. Many people who eat a Mediterranean diet aren't sitting there picking their plate trying to think if that's a calorie or not. Instead, they're having a good time, eating with their friends, and enjoying the yummy food. This diet is recognized by the World Health Organization (WHO) as a sustainable and healthy diet, and it's a cultural asset too. Remember, the focus is more on sharing these delicious meals and less on the foods you're allowed to eat and not allowed to eat.

What to Eat on This Diet

This diet wants you to frequently eat fruits and veggies, potatoes and legumes, various grains, including whole grains and breads, and some spices and herbs. You also should frequently eat seafood and use extra-virgin olive oil for cooking these foods. In moderation, you should have eggs and poultry, along with cheese and yogurt, and you should rarely eat red meat. You should only eat whole versions of these foods.

The Mediterranean Diet

This diet is a bit controversial, however. You saw bread on this list, which differs from the last two diets we looked at. The reason for such an expansive list is because so many variants exist between the countries in terms of what they eat. While you shouldn't be eating bread every single meal, you can eat bread sometimes.

The diet mostly focuses on plant foods and not as much on animal foods. However, you can eat seafood and fish in moderation two to three times a week. In general, you're allowed to have fruits, veggies, whole grains, and healthy fats every single day, at least two servings of fish a week, a weekly intake of legumes, eggs, and poultry, a limited intake of red meat, and a limited amount of dairy products. The idea behind this diet is to share it with your family and friends. You should be physically active, and yes, you can enjoy a glass of red wine with your dinner.

Wait, wine is allowed? Yep, that's right! Wine is not only allowed but has some benefits. Some wine promotes a healthy heart and is good for the body. It can even help extend your life! Make sure the wine is red because its antioxidants have the most health benefits. If you're not a fan of red, then white wine is also a good option too. If you have a history of drinking or you don't like alcohol, you do not need to drink it, but it's a nice suggestion. The Mediterranean diet focuses on treating meals as a fun experience and not something with a bunch of rules.

Meals are based around focusing on plant-based foods and not as much on meat. While you can include eggs and poultry, the seafood is often the main protein. Red meat is not eaten frequently. Another part of this diet is fats. Healthy fats are an integral part of this diet also. They're eating more of the healthy fats since saturated and trans fats cause the artery walls to thicken, and that puts you at risk for heart disease. Olive oil is one of the main sources of healthy fats, and that's because they use monosaturated fat, which lowers cholesterol levels. Nuts and seeds also have the same benefits.

Fish, especially fatty fish, is integral to this diet since they contain the healthy omega-3 fatty acids, which is great for decreasing your triglycerides, lowering the chances of blood clots, and decreasing any risk of heart failure and stroke. Fat is a good thing here. You shouldn't fear fats— just include healthy ones. Obviously, a big burger with a bunch of saturated fat should be avoided, but a nice meal of fish with steamed veggies should be something to look forward to. And don't be afraid to go nuts about nuts!

What Not to Eat

With this diet, like the others we have discussed, avoid added sugar. So beverages with sugar in them, sugars added to foods, table sugar, and even ice cream are avoided. And like other diets we discussed, you can get your sugar directly from fruits. As for grains, you can have them, but you shouldn't have refined grains. That means refined pastas, white bread, and white rice should be avoided. Trans fats are avoided, so don't eat margarine, baked goods, or other processed foods.

As for oils, you shouldn't have canola or soybean oil, and cottonseed oil should also be avoided. Whenever possible, try to use olive oil, since it's the healthiest of these oils. Processed meats are forbidden. While you should have some meat on this diet, sausages, hot dogs, and deli meats should be avoided. Highly processed foods are also restricted on this diet. Anything with a "low-fat" or similar label shouldn't be eaten. If it looks like it was made in a factory, it cannot be eaten Mediterranean style.

What Are the Pros of the Mediterranean Diet?

The Mediterranean diet is an all-around great diet, and it's a good one for many reasons. For starters, big-name science organizations have backed it. And the WHO identified it as one of the best dietary strategies for preventing and controlling non-communicable diseases and reducing premature death. This diet can help lower all causes of mortality and morbidity, and it has been linked to various health benefits, including lowering cancer, cognitive disease, and even heart disease risks.

This diet also helps with reducing inflammation in the body, which helps reduce the onset of metabolic syndrome, obesity, and type 2 diabetes. It can also help control blood sugar levels, so for those with pre-diabetes or diabetes, it can help reduce insulin resistance.

The diet is incredibly balanced, and it offers many flavors, so you won't get bored with the choices. You don't have to worry as much about whether you're overeating. This diet also benefits heart health. Your cholesterol levels and triglycerides go down, and it can help reduce blood pressure too.

While weight loss isn't the main focus of this diet, you can lose weight. That's because you're consuming less unhealthy foods, and it offers a means for you to eat whole, natural foods and reduce the bad foods. It also encourages eating more fat and less refined carbs, so you can burn the fat off the body too. The Mediterranean diet helps with energy and overall wellness levels. Many report feeling better after following this diet, and it creates balanced energy throughout the day. It can also help with insomnia. Reduced sugar intake also helps with skin health, and many report healthier skin after starting this diet.

Finally, it's environmentally friendly. You're eating foods good for you and eating less processed foods. These foods all occur naturally, and they are present in the wild. It's good for you, not hard to do, and it's good for the environment? What's not to love! This is great if you want a variety of benefits from your diet without doing a lot to achieve it.

What Are the Cons of This Diet?

This diet is great but definitely has some cons. The biggest one is cost. While this diet is great for curbing mortality in people under 65, the cost of many of these foods is much higher than with other diets, and it's hard to maintain if you're on a limited income. While there are no expensive supplements to get, this one can get pricey when you factor in the costs of the fish, seeds, and olive oil. Plus, fresh seafood is more expensive than other options.

Some conditions may also require guidance. For example, those with diabetes might need more guidance since this diet allows fruits, veggies, grain, and bread. That doesn't mean a diabetic can't benefit, but always consult your doctor before starting a new diet; for diabetics, this can be important.

It's also a bit challenging. While it isn't as restrictive as the other diets, the restrictions can make it a challenge for some people. For starters, eating less red meat and sugar is hard for the average American. There's a lot of processed sugar and foods in their diet already, and slowly reducing those takes time. It's also hard because Americans eat a lot of red meat, but you can incorporate this diet while eating smaller portions of red meat and other items.

Some get concerned about consuming alcohol, but understand that if you drink it with a balanced meal along with physical exercise, it brings many health benefits. You can enjoy alcohol safely in moderation since it can help in supporting heart health. If you are prone to alcoholism, you shouldn't consume alcohol. This is again where talking to your doctor is good.

Some nutrients are missing from this diet too. Vitamin D and calcium tend to be on the lower levels because you're not consuming enough dairy. However, there are other fortified alternatives such as almond milk, and you can eat foods such as spinach and soybeans to make up for it. If you're really concerned, try taking a supplement to help with those inadequacies.

There are no specific guidelines, such as how many calories you should have and the like. But you can put together a calorie goal that adheres to these foods and your dietary needs. Some use the USDA guidelines to build a proper meal plan that helps you get the nutrients you need. While it can be hard, sitting down with your doctor or nutritionist to work this out is usually a good thing.

Finally, it takes time. This isn't a grab-and-go diet. It requires you to prepare meals, which can be time-consuming. For those with busy lives, it requires more preparation. But once you adjust, you can learn to prepare and cook meals easily. You'll learn that preparing ahead of time, such as on a Sunday night before the beginning of the week, is the best way to go about doing this diet. It's a simple diet, but it involves some lifestyle changes and you should be willing to invest in it.

Is It Right for Me?

The Mediterranean diet is one of the easier diets to follow. While the cost can be high for some people, many people see major changes when they're following this diet.

This diet doesn't come with too many health concerns like with keto and paleo. You're still eating a balanced diet, and don't forget the wine.

It's good for those who want a generally simple diet with a few basic restrictions. Plus, if you love Mediterranean food, then this diet is perfect for you. You're eating foods they enjoy, so what's not to love.

And think about it, wouldn't a diet that involves sitting around with the family, passing around food, and having a good conversation make the diet more fun? Well, you can do that with this diet. You can build friendships around the table and enjoy food too, which is what this diet was meant for.

This diet is great because it isn't super boring and full of restrictions, and you do not have any percentage of calories or carbs to keep track of. Remember, every country has a variant of the Mediterranean diet, so you can spice it up. Maybe one week you cook a bunch of Greek food. Maybe the next Italian. The sky's the limit on what you can incorporate into the diet.

The variety of dishes you can make is another benefit. If you're a fan of cooking, you'll definitely find it easy to implement. I would recommend this diet for someone looking for a healthy lifestyle diet to lose a little weight or just maintain a well life. Someone who is diabetic or pre-diabetic may get in trouble with this diet because of the starches allowed, and people with allergies may also not like this diet because of the gluten or celiac effects.

5

DASH Diet and Whole 30

There is one silent killer that doesn't get enough recognition—hypertension or high blood pressure. Hypertension can cause many issues, including heart attacks and death. The real scary thing is you may not even know you have it, and by the time we diagnose it, you may have had it for years and it may have already affected your heart and arteries. There are ways to reverse high blood pressure via food through the DASH diet. Whole 30 is another helpful diet for underlying health issues. We'll talk about how both diets can help, and the facts behind each of them.

Overview

The DASH diet stands for the Dietary Approach to Stop Hypertension, or simply DASH. Essentially, it helps lower blood pressure in those who already have high levels or prevent high blood pressure for those at risk. So if you go to your doctor and they say, "Hey, you should probably lower your blood pressure," this is the diet for you.

This diet involves eating many different items, and it can help you lose weight. The goal is to lower your blood pressure. Losing weight may occur due to better eating habits but is not the main factor—it's more of an after-effect. It is reportedly as useful as medications that lower your blood pressure. So if you're not a fan of taking medication for lowering your blood pressure and want a more natural alternative, this could be good for you.

Essentially, they're looking to eliminate sodium from the diet. While you don't cut it cold turkey, you want to reduce your blood pressure by a few points in a couple of weeks. You can drop up to 14 points, which could put you on a different level. It's supposed to help those with blood pressure, sure, but this is also a good one for people at risk in general. For example, those who are at risk for osteoporosis, heart disease, cancer, and diabetes and stroke can benefit, since the focus is to change your diet so you're not increasing the risk for these conditions.

What to Eat

The DASH diet is simple. you can eat the following:

- Fruits
- Low-fat dairy
- Moderate grains
- Moderate fish
- Moderate poultry
- Moderate nuts

You stay away from foods high in saturated fat, so many red meats are usually out of the question. One main thing you also stay away from is high-sodium foods, usually in processed meats and the like. That's because too much sodium isn't good for you.

The DASH diet comes in two variants too, and they include:

- Eating up to 2300 mg of sodium a day
- The low-sodium version, which is where you have up to 1500 mg of sodium a day

The reason for tracking sodium is because we eat a lot more than we should. Look at any nutrition label and I'm sure you'll say "yikes" to the amount of sodium in there. Want to know how much we consume on average? About 3400 mg of sodium. It isn't good for our blood pressure and is part of the reason some people have hypertension. Cut the sodium, and you'll lower your blood pressure by a lot, which can help you.

On average, you can eat the following each day:

- 6-8 servings of grains, including rice, pasta, and cereal, focusing on whole grains since they include more fiber and nutrients.
- 4-5 servings of veggies a day, and focus on having more veggies as part of the main dish rather than a side dish.
- 4-5 servings of fruits, have them as snacks with the skin on them as much as possible since that's where the yummy nutrients are.
- 2-3 servings a day, choosing the fat-free options since this is will prevent overconsumption of saturated fat.
- 6 1 oz. servings of lean meat, fish, and poultry, since they are good for you—but too much can mean too much fat in the body and might cause your blood pressure to increase.

- 4-5 servings of nuts, legumes, and seeds, but be careful since nuts have a lot of fat content, but soy alternatives are good as well.
- 2-3 servings of fats and oils a day, but keep away from saturated and trans fats since they cause your blood pressure to skyrocket.
- 5 servings or less of sweets a week—so you can have a cookie, just don't go crazy and eat the whole jar.

What Not to Eat

You shouldn't have anything that'll make your blood pressure go up or is loaded with sodium. This may involve learning to read labels. For my patients, this is not an option, and I teach it on their second or third consultation. In general, anything processed is out of the question because if you read what's in it, you'll see the sodium levels are way too high.

Also, avoid super fatty meat. So steaks shouldn't be consumed more than once a week because they have saturated fat in them, which causes blood pressure to go up. In general, avoid trans and saturated fats as much as you can. They're not good for you and certainly won't help you lower your blood pressure.

Avoid too much alcohol and caffeine. Caffeine isn't directly discussed in the DASH diet, but it can cause your blood pressure to temporarily increase, so if you're sensitive to it, avoid it.

Try to have about 2,000 calories a day. The big thing to remember is this isn't a weight loss program. The end goal isn't weight loss, but you can lose weight while on this diet, so it's good for you.

What Are the Pros of This Diet?

The health benefits of the DASH diet are simple. There is evidence that it's proven to work. So it isn't like some of these other diets where there isn't much to go on. It reduces your risk of hypertension, stroke, diabetes, heart disease, heart attacks, and death. So yes, it can save your life. It's also pretty easy to start. After all, most of these foods are easy to get, and there are no super strict items. You just have to eat stuff that isn't super fatty.

It is flexible too. The foods to eat are suggestions, so if you want to change up something, you can. Also, this diet lets you have a sweet or two. Again, you shouldn't be binging chocolate, but if you want a dark chocolate square, you're welcome to have it. It helps you live a healthy life for a long time since it prevents many of the diseases that wreak havoc on the body.

Unlike other diets, this one has nutritional balance, so it's hard to have a nutritional deficiency. Finally, health organizations and doctors back it, so your doctor may even suggest DASH. It is good to get into the habit of eating well, and it provides lifelong wellness, which is ultimately what you should be going for.

What Are the Cons of This Diet?

Like all of our diets, this diet, too, comes with drawbacks. For starters, any convenient foods, like those frozen dinners or any quick meals, are out of the question. So if you work weird hours or can't cook, this might be hard for you to do. It requires food tracking. While it isn't strict calorie counting, it involves tracking the sodium you consume, which can be hard for some people. Some people also count calories too, which can make it tedious.

It also isn't designed for losing weight. While you can always lose weight, that isn't the end goal. The end goal is to reduce your blood pressure. Finally, this diet is overwhelming and hard to get into for some people, especially if you're a fan of shaking that saltshaker. Some people also track servings, which can get complex. So yes, it works and will help you live a healthier life. But if weight loss is the goal, it might not be for you.

What About Whole 30?

How does Whole 30 fit into this? It is a 30-day nutritional plan that encourages people to cut out grains, alcohol, sugar, additives, legumes, and dairy. It's a lifestyle challenge that can help with dieting and wellness. Nutritionists created Whole 30 in 2009, which soon became a viral sensation. Its goal is to reset the metabolism and help you build a better relationship with food. It's supposed to help you figure out which food groups affect your health and which ones are causing you the most trouble.

The diet is advertised as a way to lose weight, but really, it's good for food intolerances and finding food allergies.

What to Eat

Each week of Whole 30 involves a challenge, but in general, you can eat:

- Meat and poultry
- Fish and seafood
- Eggs
- Fresh fruits
- All veggies
- Some nuts and seeds, along with nut milk and butter
- Health plant and coconut oils

You have variants of all these foods, although you want to focus on the fresh options.

What Not to Eat

The idea is to cut out all the bad things. You're supposed to cut these out slowly, such as sugars one week, then grains the next week, then dairy and soy the next week, and then finally, beans and legumes. You can also cut all these out at once, although you may experience something similar to the keto flu or other withdrawal symptoms. The first week of this diet is by far the roughest. Most people struggle with keeping it together, and it can be hell.

Below, however, is a list of foods you can't have:

- No sugary foods or artificial or natural sweeteners, including maple syrup
- No alcohol, period
- No smoking at all

- No grains
- No legumes and beans
- No soy products
- No dairy products
- Nothing processed
- No fake "whole 30 approved" ingredients, such as paleo pancakes or cauliflower crust pizza

This might seem like a lot, but the goal is to focus on eating all of those good foods listed at the beginning and try to build a better relationship with those foods.

You eat them in their whole forms. So yes, you cook them fully and eat them as they were intended. You don't eat processed versions but just eat the chicken and veggies.

What Are the Pros of Whole 30?

This diet has many health benefits. For starters, you're cutting out sugars and other bad choices, so you will lose weight. You'll have better digestion and may have more bowel movements. Your headaches or any aches might magically improve. Sometimes we have headaches because of our diets, so it can help.

If you have acne or bad skin, your skin will clear up. You also might notice you have much more energy, and you might forgo that coffee cup. It can also help with hypertension. While hypertension is usually handled best by the DASH diet, this diet might help you if you're worried about intolerances.

It offers some new and tasty recipes, and you might crave more natural foods and less pizza. You will have better sleep, and you probably will feel a lot more energized when you wake up. It also can help with improving your blood sugar levels and curb heart disease and other problems.

However, the big benefit is to discover what foods aren't good for you. Some of us can't process grains due to the gluten. Some of us aren't good at handling sugar. Whatever is kicking your butt, the Whole 30 diet will help you find what's bothering you and creating an unpleasant experience.

You can figure out what you can't handle, and that can help a lot, especially with food allergies you might not even know exist. I tell my patients that if their arthritis is flaring, irritable bowel syndrome worsens, or they get weird rashes and headaches, it is likely from something they're eating that their body does not like.

What Are the Cons?

First, this is a fad diet. It was made by nutritionists, sure, but it's a viral diet. While it helps with figuring out any food intolerances, it is not sustainable and isn't as good for you as you think. You also are more likely to yo-yo on this diet. Yo-yo dieting is when you drop a bunch of weight only to gain it back. That happens a lot. Sure, you'll lose weight fast, but you'll get it back over time, and you might gain more.

Also, it eliminates many food groups. Sure, you should know about a gluten allergy, but eliminating these food groups also eliminates nutrients. Unless you're taking a supplement, this can pose problems in your life later. Nutritional deficiencies are quite common.

You're also getting rid of legumes, which have fiber, and unless you're eating enough veggies, you might be missing out on a ton of fiber. So you may experience more issues with constipation. But if you consume enough veggies, that can be eliminated. While ultra-processed foods aren't good, sometimes having some veggies is good to have on hand. Not all processed foods are evil—frozen foods are not bad for you. Finally, this diet is also expensive. You'll be buying a lot of fruits and veggies, and that gets super expensive. Understand this isn't for everyone.

Is It Right for Me?

Understand that the DASH diet can be sustainable, while the Whole 30 is a temporary fad diet designed to help you scope out allergies.

The DASH diet is great for those with high blood pressure or who are at risk. It can help you build healthy habits that last a lifetime. The Whole 30 diet is temporary. While it's good for figuring out food intolerances and allergies, it isn't a sustainable option. You're missing out on a ton of good foods. If you do it, consider reintroducing foods that don't affect you immediately afterward and see which ones give you trouble. You can then adjust from there.

Both can help with hypertension but in different ways.

6

Plant-Based Diets/Vegan Diets

"Eat your vegetables." That's something you've probably been told as a kid but always wondered why vegetables were so important. Did you know you can eat a whole diet based on veggies? Plant-based (vegetarian diet) and vegan diets are incredibly popular. In this chapter, we'll discuss both diets—what they are, what to eat, the pros and cons, and the bottom line.

What Is a Plant-Based Diet?

A plant-based diet involves eating food that comes from plants only. In contrast to vegetarian diets, which allow you to eat foods that come from animals, like milk and eggs, vegan diets take it a step further and cut out all animal ingredients or products. If you don't drink milk and don't eat meat products, then you're following a type of plant-based diet.

With vegan and plant-based diets, you're essentially meeting your nutritional needs by eating plant-based foods that aren't processed and don't contain refined or unrefined ingredients. You're not killing animals or eating their byproducts. Some people do this diet because it makes them feel good since they're not ethically harming animals. It also is a very effective weight-loss strategy and beneficial for overall health.

If the idea of eating plants for the rest of your days sound unappetizing, then look at the foods you can eat. The thing is, you're cutting out meat and animal products. You can still have all the plant-based products you want. Usually, when you do a plant-based or vegan diet, you're eating whole foods too. That means no refined foods or anything enriched with chemicals. It's just natural food from the earth, and it's wonderful.

What Can You Eat?

You may think the nature of this diet is incredibly boring. If you're doing it right, it doesn't have to be, but it does involve food preparation and, of course, dedication. You're making a lifestyle change. It can be scary since you're cutting out meat as well.

So what can you eat? Below is a list of all the foods you're allowed to eat:

- Fruits, including apples, figs, bananas, grapes, oranges, and strawberries
- Veggies, including lettuce, kale, peppers, collard greens, and the like
- Tubers, including potatoes of all kinds, yams, carrots, and even beets
- Whole grains such as quinoa, millet, barley, rice, wheat, and oats

- Legumes such as kidney and navy beans, cannellini beans, black beans, and lentils
- Nuts of all kinds
- Tofu
- Seeds
- Tempeh
- Whole-grain breads and flours
- Plant-based milks, such as almond milk

However, be sure to watch how many calories you consume. The more calorie-dense the food, the more they contribute to weight gain and other problems, despite this diet being plant-based. Depending on the food, you can eat plant-based and still not be healthy.

As you can see from the above list, there are still many foods you can eat on a plant-based diet. Plus, veganism is so popular these days, and because more people are doing it, there have been more creative recipes. So it's definitely a more feasible diet than it was even a few years ago. There are tons of cookbooks and recipe options too, so if you're sick of eating the same thing all the time, these cookbooks provide some great ideas!

Besides, plants are good for you. It might seem strange to base your diet on plants, but it is a viable and healthy diet when done right.

What Not to Eat

The foods off-limits depends on if you are vegan or vegetarian. With both diets, meat is out of the question— and this includes poultry and seafood, or products made from these things. Again, vegans do not eat any product that comes from an animal, to include yogurt, milk, or eggs, and even gelatin, which is found in many candies and sweets. Vegetarians may eat some of these things, but they do not eat any meat-based products. However, many people also claim a plant-based diet but eat seafood but not beef, pork, or chicken products. Since technically seafood are also animals, I would argue that is not a true plant-based diet.

What Are the Pros of a Plant-Based Diet?

Why is this so good for you? Well, there are a variety of reasons.

For starters, it can help with weight loss and many medical conditions. You're eating more fibrous foods and highly nutritious foods, so you'll have a better digestive system. Those who do a plant-based diet are much leaner, and it's very easy to keep the weight off. Some people don't even have to count calories to get this right! That's amazing, and it shows you can follow a diet without feeling like you're trapped under the burden of counting calories.

Whole and plant-based diets can help with many chronic diseases. It can help offset the risks of heart disease, type 2 diabetes, and it will lower your cholesterol and blood pressure. These silent killers can go off the radar, and you'll feel great too.

And it is good for the environment. You're putting less stress on the environment when you eat like this, and it reduces your carbon footprint. Some people feel these diets are the most "ethical" since you're not killing animals. That's up to you and your discretion. Some people see it as such; others just like it because it's fresher than other diets, and it doesn't require as many trackers as say the DASH diet, which tracks meals, or even keto, which works on counting those pesky carbs.

Your cholesterol may also decrease on this diet, and it helps with glycemic control. If you have insulin resistance, this is good for getting your blood sugar under control. It also reduces the hemoglobin A1C in those with type 2 diabetes and can help mitigate the problems that come with it. It can protect you from certain kinds of cancer.

The things you're eating contain a bunch of anti-inflammatory compounds, which protect you from free radicals galore, so you will notice it'll help you look younger and can make you feel good. Those anti-inflammatory compounds also protect you from some cancers. Plus, it can help with cognitive function and help prevent and manage both dementia and Alzheimer's disease. So yes, it can help you live an overall healthy life. This diet is also good because it can help you get your diet back on track and improve your health and wellness too.

What Are the Cons?

This diet is not for everyone. Those who aren't ready to make the commitment or realize you will be cooking at home will struggle with this one. This is one of the primary drawbacks of the plant-based diet. Many who aren't ready to cook at home and follow recipes will struggle. It also takes some discipline. You can do a plant-based diet, sure, but meat is all over, and animal products are not scarce. It can take some time, and you might struggle with the temptation that surrounds this diet. You won't just magically become a vegan easily, and it takes some discipline and self-control.

There are physical drawbacks too. For starters, you're not getting a ton of protein, so if you're looking to grow muscle or get muscular, this is a challenge on the plant-based diet. You'll have some muscle, sure, but it is lean muscle since most of the foods you consume aren't loaded with protein. It is true you will get protein from many sources of vegetarian foods—the question is how much protein. It also can create an iron deficiency. This especially happens in women, and it can cause anemia in some cases too. If you're anemic or already struggle with this, either take an iron supplement or modify the diet as needed.

Another problem is the lack of calcium and vitamin D. If you can get some milk, which is plant-based but has calcium, then great. You can get vitamin D naturally from the sun, but not calcium. A lack of both creates bone demineralization. It also puts you at a higher risk for fractures, so remember that when you're on this diet. Make sure you take a calcium supplement and go outside to get enough vitamin D.

Vitamin B12 is another nutrient that's lacking. This can put you at risk for immune system disorders, conditions, and diseases that happen in the small intestine, digestive disorders, and anemia. Vitamin B12 is usually found in meat and dairy, which you won't have as much of, so the solution is a supplement.

Finally, there is fatty acid deficiency, which is again a result of this diet. It usually comes from a lack of milk and certain protein products, such as shrimp and fish in most cases, and people usually get dermatitis and other skin conditions. It can cause scaly skin, and it increases water loss, subjecting you to dehydration. The food that gives you this is dairy, which the vegan diet nixes. So this can pose a problem. The solution is to make sure you're getting enough essential fatty acids and take a supplement as needed

This diet puts you at some risk for nutritional deficiencies, and that can pose a problem if you're older or are at risk for these conditions. But if you learn to incorporate a supplement into your diet or be sure you're eating enough of the plant-based foods that have what you need (which will take some education), you'll feel way better, and it makes this diet feasible.

Is It Right for Me?

Vegan and plant-based diets are super-effective ways to be healthy and free from many medical conditions, including obesity. You're eating all the foods you should be eating and eating less processed foods. Meat and dairy come with a lot of calories, so nixing them from your diet helps you lose weight.

As a weight loss solution, it works great, but it comes with some drawbacks. This diet isn't easy. Even with all the new and great resources available, and all the cool things you can make with plant-based foods, it's still not a simple task. It takes discipline to do it correctly, and you should understand that it comes down to you.

7

Fasting Diets

Fasting diets usually go by the name "intermittent fasting," but does it really work? Fasting diets are done for many reasons, such as religious holidays like Lent or Ramadan. However, other people adopted fasting for weight loss, and since then, it has become a very popular topic. So many self-help plans are available for fasting, and they come in many forms. They range from the "detox" diets, which supposedly involve flushing out "toxins" in the body, to even just purging for a certain period.

While there are variants, such as intermittent fasting, which can help, many of these diets don't work. Sure, they help you lose weight, but your body will yo-yo, meaning you'll gain it all back in a short while, and this yoyoing affects your metabolism. The risks outweigh the positives for detox diets, and they really can do more harm to the body than good. While some research has found benefits in intermittent fasting, long-term fasting doesn't help the body or do you any good. But we'll explore fasting here and discuss what it is, and the risks and benefits.

Overview

Fasting comes in many different forms. The safest of these is intermittent fasting, which involves the 16:8 ratio for fasting, and usually helps steadily burn off fat. This means you fast for 16 hours and eat during the eight-hour period. This takes a bit of time to get used to, and while it isn't a full-on fast, it can help you build a steady eating routine and help with weight loss. But it comes with some downsides. You must eat your calories during the feeding period, which is hard for some people. It is hard to get started, but if you stick with this, your body will adapt.

Fasting regimens also come in other forms, which aren't as stringent. Usually, they involve drinking only water, juice, or a laxative mixture. Some allow a couple of solid foods, but you shouldn't be eating a bunch of calories. This differs from intermittent fasting, where eating your calorie amount is encouraged, but it will just burn off more fat during fasting periods. Some of these are medical in nature, but others are mostly cultural and religious in nature, and they last for different amounts of time. They're not intended for you to lose weight, but instead a religious rite.

Fasting restricted to only fluids shouldn't be done for a long time. A day or two won't hurt most people, but children, those with a chronic health condition, or those who are pregnant should not be fasting. The real danger is those super long fasts, which go from three days to a month or longer. These can cause many health problems, and for many people, they can be a nightmare to deal with.

Intermittent Fasting

Again, there are many ways to do this. One way is to fast for 16 hours a day and eat all your calories during a specified time. The jury is out on this. Some studies show benefits and others show no benefits. You may know someone who this works great for, but then you tried it and it does nothing for you. Eating all your calories during a certain time frame requires preparation. It also goes against the body's normal circadian rhythm, so it is not a good long-term solution.

Another popular fast noted and published in the *Obesity* 2019 issue compared a type of intermittent fasting to a lower-calorie diet. In this study, the fasting was for a 24-hour period three days a week, and patients could eat a balanced diet on the other non-fasting days. That study found that in the fasting-but-balanced diet category, patients lost weight and had better medical markers, such as blood sugar and cholesterol, when compared to those who just did a lower-calorie diet, and they found the fasting group stuck to it longer.

The other group in this study fasted for three 24-hour periods a week. On the other days, instead of a balanced diet, they had no calorie restriction and could eat whatever they wanted. They did not do as well and lost no weight and had sometimes worse markers than before starting when compared to the fasting-and-balanced diet and the just low-calorie diet.

So even when it comes to intermittent fasting, you cannot just eat whatever you want during your non-fasting period and expect results. There still must be a diet change during the non-fasting period, or it is pointless. On the fasting days in that study, people were only allowed liquid non-high-calorie items such as water, tea, and broth. This, as we will review in the next section, is okay for short periods but cannot be a sustainable means of weight loss.

The Problem with Low-Calorie Fasting for Weight Loss

Fasting is not a viable weight loss option for many reasons. When you reduce your calorie intake, you *will* lose weight, but you'll also lose something far more important—muscle—and slow your metabolism. Muscle loss happens over time, and when your body is losing weight too fast, your body goes into starvation mode. Starvation mode doesn't help you burn fat, but instead, your body starts storing calories so you can feed your body, and you'll burn calories at a much slower weight.

Also, the weight you're losing isn't really fat. Guess what it is? Water. Water weight will come right back the second you start to eat again, and your metabolism won't be as fast, so you'll gain all that weight back and then some. If you fast in an unhealthy manner, you'll gain a bunch of weight in such a short while. Even worse, that weight you gained back will *not* be muscle unless you're hitting the gym, and even then, it's more likely to be fat.

So what's the point? There is no point in fasting for weight loss! It will kill your metabolism and do the opposite of what you expect. And that stinks! But we haven't even gotten to what else can happen when you do fast for weight loss. You can also have dizziness and some headaches, but your blood sugar will tank, so you'll feel weak. Your body will ache and your muscles will hurt. You'll also feel incredibly fatigued. If you fast for a long time, you can get anemia, a weakened immune system, or kidney and liver issues, and it can also cause arrhythmia, so it can hurt your heart health too. Fasting also causes nutrient deficiencies, including valuable vitamins and minerals, the breakdown of muscles, and diarrhea. When you also use laxatives, you're unbalancing your fluids and causing dehydration of various levels. The risks get worse the longer you fast, so if you do this repeatedly, it can cause a lot of damage.

You Don't Need to Detox

Detox diets are supposed to "cleanse" the body, but the truth is you don't need them. They will only make trouble for you. Detoxing might seem like a logical way to cure problems such as obesity and headaches, but there's no science behind any of this. You're just taking the advice of some snake oil salesman who says you should do what your body is already doing.

Remember, you were beautifully and wonderfully made. We have thousands of years of evolution under our belts. Different parts of the body do the cleaning job by getting rid of toxins—your kidneys, liver, and colon, for example. Your skin also gets rid of toxins, so why would you try to bypass what's already there? We will discuss this in more detail in its own chapter, but it was placed here also because many people consider detox a type of fasting diet.

Is This Right for Me?

Everyone agrees that fasting for long periods will not help you. It can be dangerous, and it isn't a way to lose weight long term. If you want to gain it all back, and then some, this is a great way to do it.

Intermittent fasting can work, but you must make sure you eat enough healthy foods to account for not eating during certain periods. If you like doing that, it could be a valid form of weight loss. The best way to stay healthy is to take in the appropriate calories and eat a rainbow of foods, including veggies and fruits, low-fat dairy, healthy fats, and lean protein. You are better off eating right and exercising correctly. If you aren't convinced and want to try fasting, though, it's best to talk to your doctor and find a way to fast that will not be detrimental to your health.

8

Detox Diets – Why They Should Be Avoided

Detox diets are popular because people think they will help them lose weight. But that's all they do, and only temporarily. They're not that good for you, they aren't an effective means for losing weight, and they can even be risky.

But what exactly are these detox diets? These are the pouch reset diets, the cabbage soup diet, or the broth and water only diet. They are usually in liquid form and done in hopes to reset whatever you feel is broken. This could be your gut health, your metabolism, or in many of my patients' cases, your gastric bypass pouch. Wakeup call—if you are doing it for those reasons, it will not achieve what you want. However, I will tell you when doing this diet can be beneficial and when it should be done.

Detox Diet: An Overview

Detox diets are a little different based on what kind of diet you're looking to follow. Their main goal is to supposedly "detox" the problematic toxins and cause you to reset and lose weight. Sure, you'll lose weight because all you are doing is drinking very few calories. But chances are you'll regain any substantial weight loss almost immediately. Some of these diets involve detoxing during fasts, as mentioned, some involve teas, and some involve drinking liquids only. Other versions might offer fruits and veggies as well.

They're incredibly short diets for a reason: you're not eating anything. They're not sustainable and you won't be able to stick to them in the long run unless you want to throw your body into starvation mode forever, or worse.

The Fun-Sucking Diet

Let's face it—diets generally aren't a walk in the park or that fun. But detox diets take it to the next level. You're not eating anything, and the first couple of days feel awful. Detox diets are not that safe, but the longer you plan to stay on them, usually, the riskier it gets. You'll feel weak throughout most of it.

Most people don't feel good on diets without nutrients or calories, for a good reason. Your body needs fuel, and these detox diets, while supposedly "flushing" out toxins, also make your blood sugar plummet, your muscles will ache for no reason, you'll feel lightheaded and dizzy, and fatigue and nausea are usually a part of the picture too. They can flush out your energy and your life.

Clean eating is a much better option, which focuses on eating whole foods without the processed aspects. They're good, and they give you better results than this detox diet. Detox diets tend to not be fun for many people because you're not eating anything and you do not feel like doing anything. Everyday tasks like work or playing with your kids will be a challenge. Many people are also not very pleasant to be around during this time because they're hangry. And forget about working out, often you're not even taking in enough calories to sustain bodily functions. And a good chunk of that weight you will lose isn't actually weight—it's just water and probably some waste from the body.

What Are the Cons?

I started with cons this time because this list is much longer than the pros. These diets are very limited. Some detox diets you eat nothing at all and either drink supplements or teas, or even bone broth, which has too few calories to consume long term. Others might allow you to eat some fruits and veggies, but it's rigid and it's the same thing repeatedly and can easily get boring. You just have the same detox plan for the duration of the diet. While you might have some herbs, powders, pills, or even enemas to help cleanse out the colon, usually, it's incredibly limited and you're not doing much.

Good luck exercising on these diets too. You might have some energy, but typically you won't since your calorie intake is so low. You won't be doing much if you do a detox diet. The diet varies in costs. Some of those "flat tummy teas" and the like do cost a bit. And there isn't much support either, except for the occasional online forum.

What Are the Pros?

While you won't have a long shopping list and prep work, the reason is obvious—you're not eating anything! So two stars for low cost and no prep. The only time I have recommended a diet like this one is before bariatric surgery. I put patients on a low-calorie liquid diet that still gives them nutrition to help shrink the liver and prepare the body for the massive change ahead, and this has been shown scientifically to be effective.

The other time I do a detox type of diet is when I have used and prescribed the ProLon diet, which is a cleanse to help jump-start new lifestyle changes or to rid the body of inflammatory cells and foster rejuvenated cells, with the idea you will be starting a better lifestyle choice. I have done the ProLon diet, which is a five-day cleanse, and I've seen cravings, allergy symptoms, and inflammation disappear.

This is the only cleanse with scientific research and data showing its benefits, mainly because of the proprietary blend they use for their formula. I do not work for the company or receive any benefit from them, but I want to let readers know what works and what does not work and what the scientific research shows. After all, that is the point of this book.

Is This Right for Me?

Outside of the ProLon diet, which is not a detox but could be considered a detox diet, the short answer is no. Most of those diets are snake oil products that don't do anything to help you. But here's the long answer. If the goal is to lose weight, sure, you might lose a few pounds, but you'll gain it all back. That's because those pounds you're losing aren't fat; they're just water getting flushed out of the system. It isn't a healthy means to lose weight.

Now for detox reasons, again, this diet is a waste of money and time. Your body is already naturally getting rid of these toxins no matter what kinds of foods you eat. Remember, you are fearfully and wonderfully made. Your liver and kidneys work just fine, and these toxins don't naturally build up there. So you're not getting rid of anything with these detox teas and supplements.

Anything that says they'll "detox the liver" or "cleanse" is also not accurate, since it won't help you and there's nothing to wash out. These things are a scam. Save your money; save the time. Eat a balanced diet and you'll get better results than the time you're on a detox diet.

The only time this is even worthwhile is if it prohibits high-fat and sugary foods, but you're eating whole foods instead. However, you're not sitting here starving your body in that case. That's just eating right, and it's better for you.

They Do More Harm Than Good

You may think detox diets are good for those with medical conditions. That isn't the case. They aren't good for people with certain medical issues. They don't improve your blood pressure or even your cholesterol. They also don't help the heart either. If you have diabetes, this is life-threatening, since it can create super low blood sugar, especially for those who get hypoglycemic.

The only exception is a detox diet that has a clean eating focus, and that could work for those with these conditions. Again, it's better to just eat a balanced diet without the "detox" added to it.

And the Best Diet is...

Detox diets don't have health benefits. They're fad diets. People pander them to you to make a quick buck, and they will not offer any health benefits. There are better ways to lose weight, get healthy, and have a clean body. Don't fall into the trap of detox diets.

9

The Standard
American Diet

Did you know that here in the United States, we have our own diet? Only when doing the research for this book did I realize our diet actually had a name and was recognized globally. They call it the Standard American Diet (SAD) or the Western Pattern Diet (WPD). When researching my own culture's diet, I was disgusted.

For us, the McDonald's and the Whataburgers and the plethora of restaurants and fast foods are a normal part of our daily life, but for the rest of the world, our food is the real silent killer. I will discuss it here because this book would not be complete without talking about our own diet, which, when you look at the pneumonic, is truly SAD.

Overview

This overview is coming straight from a combination of health and history sources. This diet is "rich in red meat, dairy products, processed and artificially sweetened foods, and salt, with minimal intake of fruits, vegetables, fish, legumes, and whole grains." Various foods and food processing procedures introduced during the Neolithic and

Industrial periods had fundamentally altered seven nutritional characteristics of ancestral hominin diets: glycemic load, fatty acid composition, macronutrient composition, micronutrient density, acid-base balance, sodium-potassium ratio, and fiber content. The typical American diet is about 2,200 calories per day, with 50 percent of calories from carbohydrates.

However, research states the nutritional quality of the specific foods comprising those macronutrients is often poor, as with the "Western" pattern discussed above. Complex carbohydrates such as starch are believed to be "more healthy" than the sugar so frequently consumed in the Standard American Diet. A review of eating habits in the United States in 2004 found that about 75 percent of restaurant meals consumed were from fast-food restaurants. This is what people say about our diet, and it is SAD.

What Does the Diet Consist Of?

Nearly half of the meals ordered from a menu were hamburger, French fries, or poultry—and about one-third of orders included a carbonated beverage drink. From 1970 to 2008, the per capita consumption of calories increased by nearly one-quarter in the United States, and about 10 percent of all calories were from high-fructose corn syrup. These numbers are even higher now.

Americans consume over 13 percent of their daily calories in added sugars. Beverages such as flavored water, soft drinks, and sweetened caffeinated beverages make up 47 percent of these added sugars. Additionally, excessive consumption of oils, saturated fats, and added sugars is seen in 72 percent, 71 percent, and 70 percent of the American population, respectively.

Vegetable consumption is low among Americans, with only 13 percent of the population consuming the recommended amounts. Boys ages 9 to 13 and girls ages 14 to 18 consume the lowest amounts of vegetables relative to the general population. Potatoes and tomatoes, which are key components of many meals, account for 39 percent of the vegetables consumed by Americans.

Whole grains should consist of over half of total grain consumption, and refined grains should not exceed half of total grain consumption. However, 85.3 percent of the cereals eaten by Americans is produced with refined grain, which has a longer shelf life but significantly less nutritional value. So to summarize, our SAD diet consists of:

- High fructose corn syrup
- Added sugar
- Excessive oils
- Saturated fats
- Potatoes and tomatoes
- Refined grains
- Oh, and don't let me forget about the burgers, fries, and coke

What Not to Eat?

Nothing in the diet is off the list. Part of the reason is that America is a melting pot and we have a mix of many diets. There is no food group, good or bad, that is not a part of this diet.

What Are the Pros?

The food tastes good, and it can be so good it is often addictive. The food is fast and cheap. If you are on the go and have no time to cook—or take care of yourself, for that matter—then this is the diet for you.

What Are the Cons?

Straight from the *Journal of Epidemiology* and the *Journal of Clinical Nutrition*, based on preliminary epidemiological studies, compared to a healthy diet, the WPD is positively correlated with an elevated incidence of obesity, death from heart disease, cancer (especially colon cancer), and other WPD-related diseases. It increases the risk of metabolic syndrome and may negatively impact cardio-metabolic health.

The WPD has been associated with Crohn's disease, diabetes, cancer, and obesity, but no worries. The good news is that as of 2010 when this data came out, it was not shown to be associated with breast cancer. Well, knowing the data, breast cancer is unfortunately now added to the list along with 100 other diseases, including sleep apnea, heart attack, and fatty liver disease cirrhosis.

Is This Right for Me?

Ten years ago, data showed this diet was unhealthy. The WPD is actually the worst diet you can be on, and I am embarrassed and very saddened to say this is the diet even I grew up on. How did we get here? Well, here are some historical facts. The Western diet present in today's world is a consequence of the Neolithic Revolution and Industrial Revolution. The Neolithic revolution introduced the staple foods of the Western diet, including domesticated meats, sugar, alcohol, salt, cereal grains, and dairy products. The modern Western diet emerged after the Industrial Revolution, which introduced new methods of food processing, including the addition of cereals, refined sugars, and refined vegetable oils and increased the fat content of domesticated meats.

More recently, food processors replaced sugar with the half-life of food. But this does not have to be how our story ends. We can change how we eat and choose the diet and lifestyle we want to live. We can choose to stop killing ourselves with our food choices.

10

And the Best Diet Is...

So what's the best diet for you? That's ultimately what you're going for. To start, I don't recommend fasting or detox diets. They don't work, and they will not help you lose weight. I also feel like any diet discussed here has more nutritional value than the Standard American Diet, and I do not recommend continuing to eat that diet.

But what about the good diets out there? Ultimately, it comes down to what you're willing to eat long term. How much effort and time will you put in? I feel that people have lost weight with many diets listed because it was better than the diet and lifestyle they had chosen.

If you're looking to cut your carbs and learn to control what you eat, then you might want to try keto or a variant of it. The South Beach diet might be the one you're looking for, or simple carb restriction works too.

If you want to eat more whole, natural foods without too many rules, then the paleo diet is probably what you want. Again, it comes with some nutritional drawbacks, but it might be good if you're eating too many processed foods like in the SAD.

Do you like plant-based food? If you're looking to drop weight and maintain it and will put the effort in to eat correctly, then consider a plant-based diet. It's good, and it'll help you naturally lose weight. There's no calorie counting or carb counting, but you do need to ensure you're getting enough micronutrients and not eating processed vegetarian nutrient-poor food.

If you're looking to lose weight but want to reduce your chances of hypertension and extend your life, then you should consider the DASH diet. This is a simple way to easily reduce your blood pressure points. While it requires some counting, it's still a good way to get healthy. But it's not a weight loss diet.

If you have food allergies, consider Whole 30. This can help you figure out if you are allergic to anything. But it isn't a long-term diet and isn't a healthy way to eat.

Then we have the Mediterranean diet, which is one of the best. It allows for wholesome food, fun gatherings, and, hey, wine is allowed. What's not to love? It can get expensive, sure, but it is a good diet if you're looking for something that gets to the point and is effective.

It's your choice what diet works best for your lifestyle. I will argue that your culture and genetics may also play a role as far as which diet will be the most effective. I feel the best diet is not a diet at all but a lifestyle. And some diets listed were lifestyle-based. To be healthier, you must restrict processed foods, refined sugar, and grains and ultimately eat more whole foods regardless of what diet or category they fall under, period.

As for me and my family, who I would consider healthy, we eat a combination of all of them, including WPD. I have a French creole background, so you can add gumbo and etouffee to my list also. We have had vegetarian-only meals, Mediterranean meals, and I have done low-carb. We cook most days of the week, which I think helps and in itself can prevent obesity. If we don't cook fresh vegetables, we cook frozen vegetables, which I feel is the next best thing. We only eat whole fruits, and my kids must eat two servings of fruit a day, separate from their vegetables. I often give it to them for snacks instead of goldfish crackers. We have given up most things processed in the house, including sweets like ice cream and cakes, but we do go out to eat once a week for either lunch or dinner. We have given up white rice, white bread, and processed meats, and we get our beef from a local farmer, grass-fed.

In summary, there is no one best diet. There are so many out there, and my goal was to educate you on these diets and give you the pros and cons of each. Choose for yourself what works best. If it is healthy and not processed, then it can be a good diet. Remember, it takes discipline on your end to have an effective diet, which needs to become not your diet but your lifestyle, so put your own discipline in place as well.

Resources

- https://www.healthline.com/nutrition/keto-flu-symptoms#why-some-people-get-the-keto-flu
- https://www.healthline.com/nutrition/ketogenic-diet-101#other-benefits
- https://www.healthline.com/nutrition/atkins-vs-keto#similarities-and-differences
- https://www.health.harvard.edu/staying-healthy/should-you-try-the-keto-diet
- https://www.nm.org/healthbeat/healthy-tips/nutrition/pros-and-cons-of-ketogenic-diet
- https://www.dietdoctor.com/low-carb/keto
- https://www.cooksmarts.com/articles/guide-to-paleo-substitutions/
- https://www.everydayhealth.com/diet-nutrition/the-paleo-diet.aspx#samplemenu
- https://www.verywellfit.com/the-mediterranean-diet-pros-and-cons-4685664
- https://www.verywellfit.com/how-does-mediterranean-diet-compare-to-other-diets-4685672
- https://www.eufic.org/en/healthy-living/article/the-mediterranean-diet?gclid=Cj0KCQjw2PP1BRCiARIsAEqv-pSfWWGUAOsjKsUhvrGKR-nrLjXxsyshscMQNEUdb78W8JzSXHZ2pQcaAr5qEALw_wcB

- https://www.mayoclinic.org/healthy-life-style/nutrition-and-healthy-eating/in-depth/mediterranean-diet/art-20047801
- https://www.verywellfit.com/dash-diet-pros-and-cons-3973825
- https://www.medicalnewstoday.com/articles/254836#benefits
- https://www.insider.com/bad-things-about-the-whole-30-diet-2019-4
- https://www.healthline.com/nutrition/whole-30#section4
- https://nunm.edu/2019/04/plant-based-diets/
- https://www.forksoverknives.com/how-tos/plant-based-primer-beginners-guide-starting-plant-based-diet/#gs.7rernx
- https://www.webmd.com/diet/a-z/detox-diets
- https://www.webmd.com/diet/features/diet-myth-truth-fasting-effective-weight-loss#2
- https://www.healthline.com/nutrition/paleo-diet-meal-plan-and-menu#section4
- https://www.brightwatermedicalcen-tre.com.au/health-benefits-of-the-paleo-diet.html
- https://www.news-medical.net/health/Paleo-Diet-Pros-and-Cons.aspx
- https://www.precisionnutrition.com/paleo-diet
- https://www.medicalnewstoday.com/articles/319196

Brennan, S. F.; Cantwell, M. M.; Cardwell, C. R.; Velentzis, L. S.; Woodside, J. V. (10 March 2010). "Dietary patterns and breast cancer risk: a systematic review and meta-analysis." *American Journal of Clinical Nutrition*. 91 (5): 1294–1302.

Cordain, Loren; Eaton, S. Boyd; Sebastian, Anthony; Mann, Neil; Lindeberg, Staffan; Watkins, Bruce A.; O'Keefe, James H.; Brand-Miller, Janette (2005-02-01). "Origins and evolution of the Western diet: health implications for the 21st century." *The American Journal of Clinical Nutrition*. 81 (2): 341–354.

Fung, Teresa T; Rimm, Eric B; Spiegelman, Donna; Rifai, Nader; Tofler, Geoffrey H; Willett, Walter C; Hu, Frank B (2001-01-01). "Association between dietary patterns and plasma biomarkers of obesity and cardiovascular disease risk." *The American Journal of Clinical Nutrition*. 73 (1): 61–7.

Heidemann, C.; Schulze, M. B.; Franco, O. H.; Van Dam, R. M.; Mantzoros, C. S.; Hu, F. B. (2008). "Dietary Patterns and Risk of Mortality from Cardiovascular Disease, Cancer, and All Causes in a Prospective Cohort of Women." *Circulation*. 118 (3): 230–7.

Kant, Ashima K. (2004). "Dietary patterns and health outcomes." *Journal of the American Dietetic Association*. 104 (4): 615–635.

Kesse, E; Clavel-Chapelon, F; Boutron-Ruault, M. (2006). "Dietary Patterns and Risk of Colorectal Tumors: A Cohort of French Women of the National Education System (E3N)." *American Journal of Epidemiology*. 164 (11): 1085–93.

And the Best Diet is...

Ravussin, E. Obesity. 2019. 27:50-58.

www.ingramcontent.com/pod-product-compliance
Lightning Source LLC
Chambersburg PA
CBHW020158200326
41521CB00006B/421